BEE VENOM THERAPY

THE APITHERAPY WAY TO HEALTH

FRANK SCHMIDT

Contents

ONE

BEE VENOM THERAPY

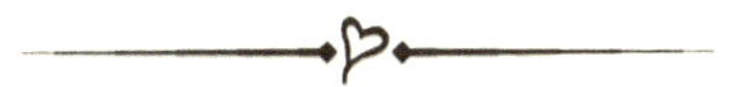

Bee venom has been given many names owing to the high number of uses it has in medicine. It can be referred to as apis mellifera, apitoxin, apis venenum, apitoxine, bee sting venom, bald-faced hornet, bombus terrestic and many others. This is the substance in bee stings which makes them painful. After years of research, bee venom has been found to contain very good healing properties and has thus been put to the use in treating autoimmune problems and chronic situations. As more research focused on this substance is undertaken, more conditions which benefit from its use are emerging. The list of the conditions that can be rectified with bee venom has significantly grown to such an extent that it is taking center-stage as one of the naturally occurring remedies that treat very many illnesses. The level of safety afforded when using bee venom is greater than what other remedies can offer. The problem has been that, all over the world, few experts are skilled in the administration of bee venom therapy. Evidence of the use of bee venom transcends across the ages as evidenced by its use in the early Egyptian and Greek civilizations to treat illnesses in human beings and animals alike. More people have invested in this natural remedy for all to benefit. The good news is that bees are everywhere and, unlike other medicines which require specific sources to work, all worker bees around the world produce bee venom.

TWO
THE APITHERAPY WAY TO HEALTH

The use of homeopathic bee venom therapy has been beneficial in Asian civilizations and European nations in the alleviation of most illnesses plaguing the population. Among the diseases that can be dealt with using bee venom therapy are multiple sclerosis, osteoarthritis, herpes zoster, carpal tunnel syndrome, Bell's palsy, neuralgias, fibromyalgia, arthritis, and many others. The fact that it is safer than other remedies has seen to a tremendous increase in the interest directed towards this remedy. However, the interest generated is not enough to show just how useful bee venom therapy is. Although people slowly recognize the fact that bee venom is beneficial to health, there is still a lot to be done to establish the benefits of this naturally occurring remedy.

What to Avoid when Using Bee Venom Therapy

here are certain foods to avoid so that the bee venom works as required. Most of these foods work in a manner that will jeopardize the effectiveness of the bee venom upon its administration. Some of these foods are common in the home and are used on a daily basis. For this reason, those with the aim of using the bee venom therapy are asked to consider having to do with these foods first. Unless the individual has other health problems which force them to feed on these foods, avoid the following foods;

- Drinks and any foods with artificial sweeteners.
- White foods such as white sugar, white rice, white bread.
- Dairy products such as sour cream, cottage cheese, cheese, milk.
- Chocolate and cocoa.
- Tobacco, cigarettes, strong tea, coffee, alcohol.
- Greasy or oily foods like fast food products, French fries, and junk foods.

The Food and Drink Products to Avoid

These foods should be avoided when one is using bee venom as a treatment therapy. The elements and compounds they contain will likely reduce the effectiveness of bee venom in the treatment process. One should also ask their medical doctor whether any other medications they are taking have these compounds and products. If the doctor states that one can still use these foods, it should be likely in small amounts to reduce their effect on the working of the bee venom.

- Drinks and foods with a lactic acid such as foxglove, tomato juice, apples, yogurt.
- Products that have been prepared from and those containing any strong aromatic oils which contain eucalyptus, peppermint, menthol or camphor e.g. candies, creams, toothpaste and others.
- Red onion, parsnips, ginseng.

- Products with sweet oils like sweet clover, sweet chervil, sweet chamomile, sweet bark, and sweet balm.
- Pops and carbonated drinks such as carbonated mineral water and most soft drinks like Pepsi Cola and Coca Cola.

What to Supplement Bee Venom With

Although bee venom is effective on its own, supplementing it with the following items will really make it more effective. The results will be realized at a faster rate since these items reduce the likelihood that the body will reject the bee venom. Also, these items will increase the rate at which the bee venom flows through the body.

- 200 to 800 mg of magnesium.
- 100 to 500 mg of vitamin B5.
- 2000 to 3000 mg of vitamin C mostly from Wampole and chewable vitamin C tablets each one at 250 mg or 500 mg.
- 2000 IU of vitamin D
- 200 to 800 IU of vitamin E
- 0.5 to 1.0 g per body weight of honey
- Propolis at three times 15-20 drops with 20 to 25% propolis tincture or 4.7 g of raw propolis. 0.5 to 0.8 g propolis tablet or capsule. One can also take propolis powder which has been mixed with honey. One should be careful to keep within 800 milligrams which is the maximum amount allowed each day. Also, avoid alcohol during this treatment.
- Bee pollen of between 7 and 15 grams per body weight
- Recommended herbs which will not work to reduce the effectiveness of the bee venom therapy.

- Royal jelly taken between 0.1 and 0.3 grams in tablet or capsule form or between 0.3 to 1.0 grams when in liquid form. It can be blended with honey or royal jelly as preferred.

What to Eat and Do when on Bee Venom Therapy

When on the bee venom treatment, one should be on a diet with high proteins. Whole foods are also advised as they enable a faster rate of healing for the body. One should be careful, however, not to include the whole foods mentioned in the list of the foods to avoid since they will reduce the effectiveness of the bee venom therapy. Sticking to the right diet and lifestyle will go a long way to ensure that the individual heals as per the requirements of their condition. The right diet entails the inclusions of foods which boost the working of the bee venom and the lack of foods which work against the bee venom.

- Each day, one should stay for at least 2 hours in an exercise program or in fresh air or both. Although some conditions may render the individual immobile, fresh air should be accessed for at least two each day.
- One should also take between 8 to 10 glasses of clean water. Water is important in eliminating toxins in the body besides allowing the body to rejuvenate from any injuries it has.
- The main sources of whole foods include whole grains, butter, seeds and nuts, eggs, cod liver oil, fish, liver, poultry, dried foods, vegetables and fruits, and many others. One should eat as much of whole foods as possible. The results will be amazing on the body since whole foods work in line with the bee venom for the very best of results.

Preparation before Using Bee Venom in Treatment

Before one delves into the use of bee venom to treat their condition, there are a few items to put into consideration to increase the effectiveness of the bee venom therapy. Rid the body of medications like steroids and non-steroidal anti-inflammatory drugs (NSAID) for at least two months although three months is the recommended period. Generally, the longer the interval one goes for without drugs in their body, the better the bee venom therapy will work. However, be careful only to stop using these indications if the medical practitioner who prescribed the medicine has agreed on this issue. Otherwise, the patient may be in trouble for deserting their medication. It may require long periods of consultation with skilled and knowledgeable people on this subject to decide if it is right for the patient finally.

THREE

THE CONDITIONS WHICH CAN BE REMEDIED WITH THE BEE VENOM THERAPY

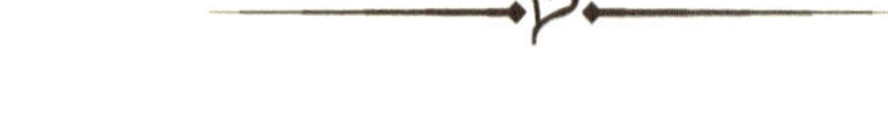

There is a long list of illnesses that can benefit directly or indirectly from bee venom. Also, one can get the bee venom either directly from live bees, or through using a homeopathic solution of bee venom such as Apex Venenum Purum which is approved by the FDA for safety and effectiveness of use in dealing with certain conditions. Following extensive research, the most knowledgeable minds on the use of bee venom have all agreed that these conditions can be helped with this solution.

Allergies

The field of allergology has concluded that the allergic reactions to bee venom can be done away with using a continuous administration of this venom below the skin. With time, the individual is desensitized to bee venom as evidence has shown. The amount of bee venom should be small at the beginning and rise as the individual becomes more desensitized.

Cardiovascular diseases

In cardiology, bee venom can be used to help prevent and treat these diseases;

I. Acute rheumatic fever
II. Arthritis obliterans
III. Arrhythmias
IV. Arteriosclerosis
V. Coronary heart diseases
VI. Atherosclerotic arthritis of the inferior limbs
VII. Hypotension
VIII. Peripheral ischemia degenerative syndrome
IX. Reynaud's disease

In most cases, however, bee venom may be combined with other types of medications or remedies that work in line with it. However, bee venom has been proven to be effective on its own.

Endocrine System Diseases

Bee venom has severally found use in treating various issues with the endocrine system which is responsible for the secretion of hormones and other substances in the body. The body may not be action as required by, for example, producing too little or too much of a certain hormone or hormones. Bee venom therapy will correct that. The diseases treated by bee venom include;

· Hyperthyroidism

- Cortisol secretion dysfunction
- Hypoglycemia
- Menstrual cramps
- Irregular menstrual periods
- Premenstrual syndrome (PMS)

Rheumatologic Diseases

Many of the diseases that plague the skeletal system can immensely benefit from the use of bee venom therapy. They include;

- Articular rheumatoid diseases such as rheumatoid, gout, traumatic gout, osteoarthritis, and psoriatic.
- Non-articular rheumatoid diseases such as tendonitis, bursitis, scars, fibromyalgia and Dupuy tren's contracture.

Pulmonary Diseases

The pulmonary system will benefit immensely from the use of bee venom therapy. Among the ailments taken care of by this remedy are;

- Emphysema
- Chronic obstructive pulmonary disease
- Asthma

Neurological Diseases

The nervous system is not left behind when it comes to the benefiting from the bee venom therapy. The neurological diseases treated by bee venom include;

- Cerebral thrombosis
- Chronic pain syndrome

- Dupuytren's contractors
- Lumbago neuralgia
- Zona-zoster
- Bell's palsy
- Multiple sclerosis
- Post-herpetic neuralgia
- Neuritis, sciatica
- Guillain-barre syndrome
- Neuralgias
- Carpal tunnel syndrome
- Diabetic neuropathy

Skin Diseases

In dermatology, it has been widely agreed that bee venom helps alleviate a lot of problems that people suffer from. The list includes;

- Degranulated wounds
- Bruises or the blue skin contusion
- Hair loss
- Low sensitivity
- High sensitivity
- Lupus erythematosus
- Moles
- Melanoma
- Mycosis fungoides
- Psoriasis
- Eczema
- Tropical ulcers
- Scars
- Skin tumors and vascular skin tumors

Immunological Diseases

Problems that plague the immune system also get treated using the bee venom therapy. The list of the diseases under this consideration includes the following;

- AIDS
- Endarteritis obliterans
- B-Cell enhancement
- Lupus Erythematosus
- Scleroderma
- T-Cell Suppression
- Systematic Lupus Erythematosus

Infections

Bee venom can be used to do away with infections of various types such as;

- Viral meningitis
- Shingles
- Warts
- Mononucleosis
- Chronic fatigue syndrome
- Epstein-Barr disease
- AIDS

Psychological Diseases

There is a long list of psychological disease that can be treated using the bee venom therapy. Many of the diseases in this list may be similar to those included in the list of the neurological disease. However, purely psychological problems include the following;

- Anxiety
- Depression

- Substance abuse

Conditions Which Make Using Bee Venom Problematic

There are some contra-indications which must be put into consideration to ensure that the bee venom does not work against the body's working mechanisms. They include the following;

- Cardiac insufficiency
- Bee venom allergy
- Kidney insufficiency
- Local and systematic infections
- Pulmonary insufficiency
- Feverish diseases
- Pregnancy
- Purulent infections
- Unwillingness to use the venom
- Insulin dependent diabetes
- Liver cirrhosis
- Digestive ulcers
- Under prescription for beta-blockers as bee venom works antagonistically to beta-blockers such as epinephrine which will have little efficiency during anaphylactic reactions.
- Lung diseases such as advanced lung insufficiency or tuberculosis
- Kidney insufficiency such as albuminuria, nephritis, glomerulonephritis, polycystic kidneys and others.
- Any severe psychiatric conditions such as anxiety, psychosis, and depression.
- Do not use bee venom right before or right after a meal.
- Bee venom should not be administered to children under 12 years of age.

- When breastfeeding, avoid bee venom.

Deciding on Bee Venom Therapy

- Given that bee venom may be a relatively new section of medicine to some people, there are factors one can put into consideration to ensure that they make the right decision on this medical remedy.
- First of all, one should consult with their medical doctor to determine the available options for treatment be they holistic or conventional.
- One should also focus on doing personal background searches to establish the suitability of this remedy. Among the items to focus on include the limitations of this remedy, its side effects, and the outcomes of the treatment. There are many places to search for information including local libraries and apitherapy research centers. However, the internet will provide lots of important information on this subject.
- Consider also what is consistent with one's belief system. It is understandable that some people may find it hard wrapping their minds around the concept that painful bee stings are being used as medicine. However, further research into what the bee stings have in terms of their chemical composition will lead to a better understanding of this naturally occurring remedy.
- It should also be considered whether the individual is ready to follow a routine which does not involve drugs but focuses only on vitamins, supplements, avoiding certain foods and exercise routines. Some find it too unconventional to stay away from certain drugs and fully adopt the bee venom therapy. The changes being suggested may be permanent such that one may be fully

weaned from some drugs.

- Consider, also, the side effects that may come from the use of this remedy should be considered to ensure that the individual is ready to live with them.
- The cost of the therapy should be on the checklist before adopting this therapy. For most people, using the bee venom therapy may come across as an expensive method. Consulting with the medical practitioner goes a long way in ensuring one is financially ready to take on bee venom therapy.
- It is clear that bee venom therapy may require people to stay away from certain types of foods for the long term. One ought to be ready to know that they may just be giving up their favorite dish for good. Either way, using bee venom for treatment is not a strict a dieting method as other remedies which may require total abandonment of certain foods. For example, using insulin injections requires that the individual stays clear of sugar since their body cannot naturally control it.
- The injections for bee venom therapies are between two and three for each week. If one is psychologically ready to have themselves pricked for this amount of injections over a given period of time, they are ready to have this type of therapy.
- After deciding to undergo the bee venom therapy, one should consult with their doctor to establish whether they will ditch or continue with their current medications as there are some medicines which do not work with bee venom well.
- The medical practitioner administering the medicine should be ready to monitor the progress of the treatment to ensure that it is safe and there are no incidences of unexpected issues. Monitoring is very vital

in bee venom therapy as it allows the medical doctor decide whether the venom is working as required or not. If, also, there are any cases of allergic reactions and other side effects.

- If one decides not to undergo the bee venom therapy, they should inform their medical practitioner so that they are allowed to continue with their prevailing medical routine.

Methods of Obtaining and Applying Bee Venom

1. **From live bee stings**;the bees to be used for this treatment are stored away from the hive for a certain period of time. Their stings are then applied to acupuncture points or on other tender points to enter the body. The stings can be applied using acupuncture needles of alone. Although often said to be the most effective method, using bee stings directly is subject to the location where the bees were harvested from and their breed. The reason direct bee stings are touted to be the best method is that storing bee venom is a difficult process owing to the volatility of the venom when outside the body of the bee.

2. **Bee venom cream**; the bee venom is harvested from the bee stings and made into a cream which is applied to the skin between 2 to 3 times per day.

3. **Bee venom injections**;the venom is harvested from the bees without necessarily killing them. It is then stored in ampoules where is it diluted with an anesthetic to make it painless. The injections are made on the tender parts of the body.

Noted Reactions to Bee Venom

The use of bee venom has been proven to be very safe especially when prepared and administered well. For the most part, they are the normal reactions to a bee sting but toned down so much that some patients rarely feel anything at all. In the reactions that occur, there could be some itching, heat, mild swelling and some redness on the area of the injection. There is nothing wrong with these reactions as they are what is expected of the injections. They may last a few days to 5 days and go away on their own due to their self-limiting nature. Some cases have reported symptoms similar to these noted in flu, but they still go away after a few days. One should be aware that such reactions are signs that, indeed, the body is fighting through the introduced venom. All that is needed is observation. However, if one notes any other abnormal signs, they should call their medical doctor as fast as possible. Also, one can take several measures to do away with the discomfort caused by the bee venom injections. For example, taking lots of supplements and vitamins has been proved to increase both the effectiveness of the venom, and reduce the level of discomfort caused by the venom on the body. One can also use a soft brush to massage the area that is itchy in order to provide relief for a given period. Rough materials should be avoided as they are likely to cause damage to the skin besides swelling and increased soreness. The application of Preparation H Cream which is an anti-itch cream with hydrocortisone 1% on the areas of the skin where the injections or stings have been administered should relieve the pain and itch from the areas. In some cases, using a meat tenderizer (in small amounts) on the injected area reduces the pain. Be warned, however, that the meat tenderizer has been proven to reduce the bee venom's effectiveness. It should thus be avoided as much as possible and only used as a last resort. The patient should avoid the use of NSAIDs such as Tylenol, Naprosyn, and Motrin besides antihistamines, Benadryl and Calamine as they all work against the bee venom and thus reduce its effectiveness.

The Safety Level of Bee Venom

Many people erroneously compare bee stings to the wild tales they have heard about bees killing people and yet, the same bee stings are being advertised as medicine. Scientific findings have portrayed a different picture altogether. First of all, bee venom is among the safest natural remedies on the planet. For an adult of weight 166 lbs, at least 1425 bees stings are needed to be termed lethal and kill them. For a child of 66 lbs, at least 570 bee stings are needed to make a lethal dose. There are cases of people who have survived at least 1000 bee stings on their bodies. Even better is the knowledge that bee venom has a very high ratio of medicines to toxins. The ratio is at 70 while most medicines have a value of less than 10.

Very few cases of severe allergic reactions. Only 1 in every 150,000 people have the risk of anaphylactic reactions. That is indeed good news as it shows the likelihood of deaths and allergic reactions is very low. The individual administering the bee venom, however, needs to have Benadryl or EpiPen at the ready to make sure that they take care of any emergency that may arise. In most people, however, the reactions to the venom are mostly mild.

How Bee Venom Works

How can venom be used as medicine? One may ask. Worker bees produce the venom in a special sack with the intention of keeping off predators from invading the colony. The queen in the hive has also been known to produce venom. Her's, however, is more of a self-defense mechanism than for the hive as she kills her competition with it. The properties of bee venom set it aside from the stings of insects such as hornets and wasps as people respond differently to each sting.

Besides activating the immune system, bee venom has many benefits in the body including its anti-oxidant effects, reducing inflammation and pain, stimulating the pituitary-cortisol all system, improving the flow of blood, improving the body's level of strength, and the conversion of chronic conditions into acute ones. The table below details the common drugs from bee venom, how they act, and their effects.

Evidence and Research on Bee Venom

Among the reasons science has shown considerably low interest in bee venom is that potential researchers and investors see no value in it as one cannot patent a remedy that occurs in abundance naturally. For this reason, they see no profit potential in bee venom as a medicine. The result of this low level of interest has seen to the lack of investments in the research into bee venom. Lastly, few other substances with properties such as bee venom exist. For this reason, the tests on humans are mostly in their trial phases for the very advanced medical conditions. It thus upon the consumers to determine whether they will use bee venom or not given that the findings at hand are from clinical observations, case studies and case reports under uncontrolled environments. Although there is a lot of interest generated in bee venom all across the globe, the most active nations in this regard are Japan, China, and South Korea where a lot of funds have been injected into the research of this chemical. The medical field anxiously awaits these findings to know the real potential of bee venom on the health of humanity.

Historical Background on All Bee Products

For a very long time, products from the hive have been used by generations of people. 2400 years ago, Egyptians and other civilizations were already using products from their bee hives. Evidence of this can be seen in the pictures and other findings in all cultures across the ages. The medical fraternity swears by the Hippocratic Oath to always protect the life of their patient at any cost. The owner of the name, Hippocrates, has been touted to the father of modern medicine. In his works, Hippocrates used honey and other beehive products with excellent results. Another notable medical person in history is the Roman physician Galen who is said to have been prescribing honey for all purposes. A look at the art from ancient Mayan and Aztec carvings depicted the popularity of bees and beehive products. Alexander the Great is also often said to have widely employed bee venom therapy after his endeavors on the battlefield. Charlemagne, who built the famous Palatine Chapel of Charlemagne and built a vast empire in present-day Germany, got rid of his gout using bee venom therapy. Philip Terc, the famous physician of the 1800s, had a very impressive enough record treating patients of arthritis with bee venom. Besides honey and bee stings, the hive offers other useful products such as bee pollen, propolis, and royal jelly which have wide applications in the medical field. The products are in use all over the world. The products include;

1. **Royal Jelly;**also called honeybee milk, royal jelly is what makes up a majority of the food of the queen bee. Royal jelly makes the queen both energetic and highly fertile. Royal jelly is derived from the young worker bees which are between 4 to 12 days old. They feed the queen bee with their milk but grow up and stop producing the milk. For this reason, Royal jelly is very hard to come

by in a hive. When obtained, honeybee milk is used in the treatment of a one list of ailments among them hyperlipidemia, arteriosclerosis, metabolic diseases, chronic kidney insufficiency, lack of or too little sexual hormones, adrenal gland disease, and menopause. Although it has not been proven by science yet, royal jelly has been related to increase in the lifespans of those who use it. However, there are some health conditions that will not permeate the individual to use royal jelly. They include allergies, acute cancer, and acute bronchial asthma. Owing to its unstable nature, royal jelly needs to be stored as a mixture with other items like propolis or honey, or it can be frozen to remain stable. China is the major work exporter of royal jelly, and it exports tons of the compound each year.

2. **Bee Pollen;**when bees collect honey from trees and plants, they go for the protein the pollen with which they feed their young ones with. The bee pollen contains very many nutrients such as minerals, vitamins, and some essential amino acids. The way bee pollen is, it has many properties to heal the body in several important ways. It can be used as an anti-allergen, anti-toxin, antioxidant, antidepressant, antibacterial, anti-atherosclerotic, and even as an aphrodisiac. It has also been found to reduce the level of stress in users besides reverting the blood pressure to normalcy. The immune system can also immensely benefit from bee pollen, and so does the stomach, large intestine, and the thyroid. Its use as an aphrodisiac also transcends into its use in the improvement of the prostrate. Generally, bee pollen affords the body energy and a good feeling by its activation of various items in the body. Its contribution to the increase in the number of red blood cells in the

body cannot go unmentioned. The normal bee pollen dosage starts with a few grams before increasing to between 1 and two teaspoons each day. To increase its healing properties and absorption rate, bee pollen is mixed with honey.

3. **Propolis;** bees collect propolis in the securing of the hive and the protection of the colony from being infested with microorganisms such as parasites and bacteria. Bees collect this substance for the backs and buds of trees. The propolis has various properties such as being a local anesthetic, a stimulant for the immune system, anti-tumor, antiviral, anti-stress, antiseptic, anti-oxidant, anti-edema, anti-inflammatory, anti-herpetic, anti-hemorrhage, anti-allergic, antibacterial and as an antidepressant. Cancer patients also use propolis to reduce the side effects of radiotherapy and chemotherapy by protecting the body against radiation and stimulating the regeneration of tissues in the body. Propolis should not be used by those allergic to it and those with a low blood pressure. On the outside of the body, propolis is used as toothpaste, shampoo, cream, and as drops. Internally, it is used as a tablet, syrup or tincture.

FOUR

FINAL THOUGHTS

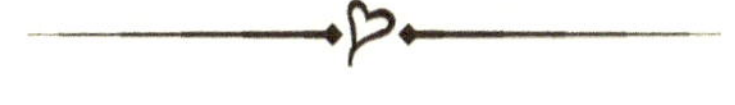

While many people find it difficult accepting the fact that venom can be used a form of medicine, it ought to be known that many poisons in nature contain a lot of medicinal properties. For example, aloe vera is a very bitter plant in terms of the taste of its extract is concerned. In fact, there are plants in the same family as aloe vera that are purely poisonous. Even animals such as poisonous snakes have their poisons extracted and made into some very important medicines for use across the board.